Doctors vs. Nurses

Collaboration vs. Chaos

The Theory of Mutual Respect and Collaboration

Kamran Hasni, MD and Mary Perkins RN, MSN, MHA

DISCLAIMER

The medical information provided in this book is, at best, of a general nature and cannot substitute for the advice of a medical professional.

This book is designed to provide information and motivation to our readers. It is sold with the understanding that the publisher is not engaged to render any type of psychological, legal, or any other kind of professional advice. The content of this book is the sole expression and opinion of its authors, and not necessarily that of the publisher. No warranties or guarantees are expressed or implied by the publisher's choice to include any of the content in this volume. Neither the publisher nor the individual author(s) shall be liable for any physical, psychological, emotional, financial, or commercial damages, including, but not limited to, special, incidental, consequential, or other damages. Our views and rights are the same: You are responsible for your own choices, actions, and results.

Names, characters, businesses, places, events, and incidents are either the products of the author's imagination or used in a fictitious manner. Any resemblance to actual persons, living or dead, or actual events is purely coincidental.

This book is dedicated to all patients, nurses, and doctors who work towards mutual respect and collaboration.

CONTENTS

	Acknowledgments	i
	Preface	iii
	Introduction	v
1	Why Should We Care?	1
2	Are We One of the Statistics?	5
3	Then and Now: History of the Health Care Dynamics	8
4	The Dynamics of the Theory of Mutual Respect and Collaboration	14
5	Respect	64
6	Collaboration	72
7	Resolution	78
8	Future of Health Care	87
9	The Theory of Mutual Respect and Collaboration	90
	About the Authors	94

Copyright © 2013 Hasni Publishings

All rights reserved.

ISBN: 1494318105
ISBN-13: 978-1494318109

Original cover design by Julie Burnette

ACKNOWLEDGMENTS

We would like to thank the many people who helped make this book happen. To our editor, Sandra Stevens. To our project manager Maria Swafford. Also, thank you to Julie Burnette for all the cover designs and photography.

PREFACE

The dynamics involved in patient-nurse-physician relationships are vital forces that affect the outcome of the health of the patient both directly and indirectly. The traditional roles of patient, nurse, and physician have always involved a clearly understood hierarchy in which the doctor was the apex, the nurse the intermediary, and the patient the base of the health care pyramid.

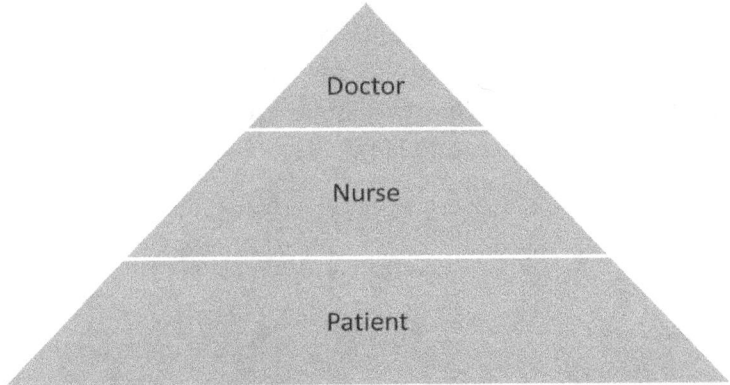

In recent years this once strictly delineated hierarchy has changed substantially, and those who hold the traditional view are becoming a disappearing minority. The necessity for and availability of health care related information has increased dramatically for everyone involved in the designing, implementing, and assessing of health care plans. Thanks to mandatory public education and the internet, today's patients are more knowledgeable and more likely to want to take an active role in their plan of care than patients were in the past. Nurses are now required to obtain and maintain a much more extensive education and are held accountable for their actions in the care of patients. Doctors now focus on increasingly specific specialties and can find out about the latest medical breakthroughs almost as soon those breakthroughs are made.

The Theory of Mutual Respect and Collaboration has been developed to bring a better understanding of the need to re-shape the health care hierarchy from a strict three layered pyramid into a synergistic, convex shaped pyramid that is formed at the center of three overlapping spheres. Each intersection of spheres would equate to one of the key dynamic health care relationships: patient-doctor, patient-nurse, or doctor-nurse. In this version collaboration is the glue that holds the spheres together. The small center pyramid is the "sweet spot" that leads to optimal patient care.

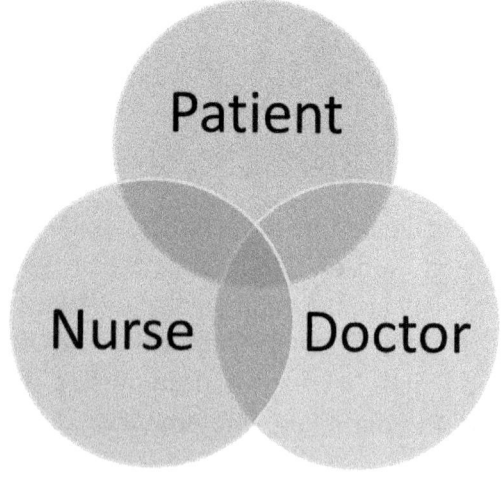

INTRODUCTION

"Patient Has Wrong Limb Amputated", "Young Teen Dies When Given Wrong Medication", "Doctor Sued for Malpractice - Blames Nurse", "Nurse Says She Told Doctor Chart Was Wrong", "Nurse was 'Just Following Orders' – Child Now Paralyzed"

Anyone who is in health care has heard horror stories about a patient having the wrong limb amputated because of a miscommunication, or a patient dying because of an allergic reaction to a drug that was listed as an allergy on the patient's chart. Imagine an even worse scenario of a patient who suffers injury or death as a result of the arrogance in judgment of a nurse or physician. Now imagine that this could be one of your own family members, or even you. Even though health care providers do not associate themselves with these alarming statistics, the truth is physicians and nurses will be patients themselves at some point in their lives. How would you want your physician and nurse to communicate with each other? Obviously you would want open communication and honesty to be a priority in the care being provided to you and your family. A nurse or doctor who disregards information provided by a patient or other health care providers would not only be acting disrespectfully but could be acting dangerously. A nurse who is so afraid to offer information to a physician perceived as unapproachable is still accountable when the lack of that information leads to poor care, injury, or possibly even death. These are important factors all health care providers must keep in mind. When physicians and nurses assume care of patients, they owe it to their patients to give them the best quality care possible; after all that is why they became health care professionals isn't it?

1. WHY SHOULD WE CARE?

The number of people having in-hospital, adverse reactions to prescribed drugs annually: approximately 2.2 million. (1)

The number of unnecessary and/or inappropriate antibiotics prescribed annually: approximately 45 million per year. (2)

The number of unnecessary medical and surgical procedures performed each year: 7.5 million. (3)

The number of people unnecessarily hospitalized each year: 8.9 million. (3)

If these estimates are correct, then there are more than 2,216,000 serious adverse drug reactions (ADRs) in hospitalized patients, causing over 106,000 deaths annually. These statistics do not include the number of ADRs that occur in ambulatory settings. Also, it is estimated that over 350,000 ADRs occur in US nursing homes each year. (3)

According to the CDC, in American hospitals alone, healthcare associated infections account for an estimated 1.7 million infections and 99,000 associated deaths each year. (4) The most stunning statistic however, is that the estimated total number of iatrogenic deaths- that is, deaths induced inadvertently by a physician or a surgeon or by medical treatment or diagnostic procedure in the US annually is at least 794,936. It is evident that the American medical system is itself the leading cause of death and injury in the US. By comparison, approximately 652,091 Americans died of heart disease in 2005, while 559,312 died of cancer. (5) A report states that in one decade there were 8 million deaths caused by conventional medicine. (6) ("Hospitals May Be Hazardous To Your Health", 2013). The mortality costs alone exceed $282 billion a year.

The National Coalition on Healthcare reports that annual healthcare spending in the US has been increasing two to five times the rate of inflation since 2000. (7) Total healthcare spending was $2.4 trillion in both 2007 and in 2008, or $7,900 per person, which represented 17 percent of the gross domestic product. (8) The total is projected to reach $3.1 trillion in 2012. (9) That's about 4.3 times the amount spent on national defense. (10).

These alarming facts force the health care industry to take notice of how patient care is communicated between providers. There is a realization that the communication between the physicians, nurses, and patients has to change in order to provide safe, effective care to patients.

Although healthcare has greatly changed in the way these relationships are viewed, there is still a long way to go. For this reason, a Theory of Mutual Respect and Collaboration needs to be utilized in order to cultivate a new culture in health care where the dynamics involved in the communications between patient, nurse, and physician are based on collaboration with each other and respect for each other's contributions to the plan of care.

When the dynamics fail to work together the results can become deadly. The chaos of September 11, 2001, clearly showed that people not collaborating with each other can have devastating results. This is an extreme case of failure to communicate, but it proves the point that chaos can ensue if collaboration is not used in any area. Just as each agency involved on that day shouldered some fault for not sharing information with others, so are healthcare providers responsible for collaborating with each other in order to have a better patient outcome. If the agencies had shared and accepted each other's input, then many of the 3,497 people who died in that tragedy might still be alive today. The government identified the problem and has since worked on ways to have more communication and collaboration between the agencies. The health care field needs to do the same. Now healthcare has identified that poor communication and lack of collaboration have been a long existing problem. As health care changes it is crucial for nurses as well physicians to lay aside their own egos and work together to offer the best outcome possible for the patient. This means developing effective collaboration that includes the doctor, nurse, and patient establishing a culture of respect and motivating all concerned to work together to find the best outcome possible.

2. ARE WE ONE OF THE STATISTICS?

Problems with communication and collaboration have also plagued the healthcare field for many years, and despite many other advances, these problems still exist today. According to one report from the Institute of Medicine, up to 98,000 deaths occur in one year because of medical errors. The report also indicates that many fatalities are directly related to miscommunication. This makes us ask ourselves, "Could we be one of the statistics?" If we are not open to communication and collaboration, the answer is "Yes, we are one of the statistics."

As health care changes, it is crucial for nurses and physicians to lay aside their own egos and work together to offer the best outcome possible for the patient. Patients must also learn how to become effective partners in developing and following effective healthcare plans. A healthy collaborative approach by the physician, nurse and patient will result in the best outcome possible.

In a 2000 study, Sexton et al. asked members of an operating room and aviation crew similar questions about culture, teamwork, and hierarchies. While attending surgeons perceived that teamwork in their operating rooms was strong, the rest of the team members disagreed, proving that one should ask the followers, not the leader, about the quality of teamwork. Perhaps more germane to the patient safety question, while virtually all pilots would welcome being questioned by a coworker, or subordinate, nearly 50% of surgeons would not. (11) In a 2011 study, while these differences in perceptions among surgeons, anesthesiologists, and nurses had narrowed somewhat, they had not gone away.

The goal of this book is to help all those involved in healthcare, including the patient, to form strong collaborative partnerships. The presentation of various narratives and scenarios that describe healthcare experiences of patients, nurses, and physicians will provide insight as to how each person or partner involved perceives the others' contributions to the plan of care. Analysis of the situations will aid readers' understanding of how each partner can help change the culture of health care. Understanding the Theory of Mutual Respect and Collaboration will help nurses, physicians, and patients work more collaboratively to improve the communication and delivery of healthcare which will reduce the number of medical errors and increase the effectiveness of health care plans.

The Theory of Mutual Respect and Collaboration focuses on the three main contributors to the dynamics in a patient's plan of care. This is not to ignore the contributions made by other health care providers such as respiratory therapists, aides, counselors, etc. as their roles are also important. The three focal points of concern in this theory are the patient, nurse, and the physician because the dynamics involved in their relationships are often the sources of miscommunication and poor decision making that lead to feelings of inadequacy and resentment, and too often result in lowering the quality of care a patient receives. At the root of most negative relationships is a lack of trust and respect between the individuals which often leads to a failure to communicate effectively. The scenarios in this book will further illustrate the effect that disrespect and lack of collaboration have on the overall plan and quality of care provided. In this environment relationships become distrustful and possibly antagonistic; it is doctors versus nurses versus patients, and chaos is a common result.

3. THEN AND NOW: HISTORY OF THE HEALTH CARE DYNAMICS

Historically the roles of the patient, nurse, and physician were clearly understood by everyone involved including the patient's family and friends. The patient was the one in need of care. If first aid or home remedies provided by friends and family or initiated by the patient did not work, the patient would then seek the services of a physician. The physician's job was to diagnose the problem or disease, prescribe medicines, and provide instructions regarding patient care. Usually one of the patient's family members would be pulled aside and given the orders in detail. This family member served as the patient's nurse. Whether at home or in a hospital, the patient had one role – take the medicines prescribed and follow the orders of the physician and the nurse. The nurse's role, again whether working with a patient at home or in the hospital, required the nurse to follow the doctor's orders and provide appropriate care as ordered by the doctor. A closer examination of each of these roles will help us understand the historical basis of these relationships and the reasons the underlying assumptions and perceptions need to change.

Until relatively recently, patients' medical knowledge was limited to stories and recipes handed down within their family or community. Even as more and more people became literate, this did not include any reliable medical knowledge. Doctors often had to combat both patient and family ignorance or misunderstanding about health practices, such as adding heat to a feverish patient. Then, as is also true now, the patient made the final decision; if the patient did not understand the directions, did not trust the doctor, or would not follow the nurse's orders, the whole plan of care could quickly become ineffective. The efforts of all involved would be wasted. To simplify things, physicians usually focused on the dangers of not following orders and not on educating the patient as to the causes of illness or detailed effects of the medicines or procedures. Since most patients were illiterate at that time, they had little recourse but to do as told or stay sick or maybe even die.

In the hospitals, paid nurses took care of patients. Nurses were traditionally expected to be young, unmarried, and devoted to serving the patient, as well as the physician. The expectations for being a nurse were simply to be able to work hard, be subservient to the physician, and care for the patient. Other helpful qualities were to be tall, clean, neat in appearance, and to have the ability to please the patient and physician. Some of the historical qualifications even went so far as to say a nurse should have a good figure and have good looks, as well as well as being able to play tennis, ride horses, and dance, as it was thought that these qualities would help the nurse move with finesse in the wards of infirmaries. Nurses never dreamed of questioning a doctor's orders and focused on making sure the patient did exactly as the physician expected. Since patients in a hospital knew they were at the mercy of the nurse for not only medical care, but also for their most basic needs – food, water, and clean bedding, they usually were quite compliant. Nurses had to tread a fine line; they were in charge of the patient, but were responsible for making sure the patient followed orders. Doctors in hospitals had little time for lengthy discussions with either nurse or patient; they relied on nurses to understand what was needed and see that it got done.

Traditionally in America, doctors were male and often were single. They were considered the authority on the care of patients, and their orders were carried out without question from the nurse or the patient. While formal education of medical doctors was sporadic, the profession did demand a lot of time and dedication. Most doctors received training via a relatively long apprenticeship from another doctor. Since doctors were not licensed, the quality of this type of education varied greatly. However, compared to other members of the community, they were exceptionally skilled and knowledgeable. They were greatly respected if not highly paid, and in addition to serving as physicians often held positions of leadership in their communities.

It is easy to understand why doctors grew accustomed to having others look up to them. When it came to developing a plan of care for a patient, it was totally the doctor's responsibility to decide what medications, procedures, and strategies would be used, as well as how and for how long they would be used. No one was in position to question his medical decisions.

A great deal has changed since then. One main difference in the roles of the patient, nurse, and physician of today is that the knowledge base of all three has increased dramatically. Most patients are literate to some degree, and they have access to more information. Public libraries, mandatory Kindergarten through 12th grade education, and the internet make information not only easy but cheap. As a result patients often research their own health problems and disease processes. They find that there may be more than one option for treatment. Now, the patients often insist on being active participants in their plans of care; they no longer just accept the information of one physician. Patients are getting second opinions and seeking alternative therapies to their diseases.

Qualifications for being a nurse in today's healthcare field is based on completing an accredited nursing program and maintaining the credentialing required by the state in which they practice. Nurses can earn degrees from the associate to doctorate level. Nursing qualifications are based on education not looks. Some things that haven't changed are the requirements that nurses have compassion for their patients and be able to interact with the patient and physician; however, the difference is that this interaction takes place on a more professional level. Nurses have fought to be able to govern themselves and have established nursing as a profession; it is no longer a menial task-focused job. Nurses have to complete strenuous courses of study and pass state board exams in order to be licensed. Nursing has legitimized the profession with advanced degrees and varied fields of study. Nurses now can be independent practitioners, administrators, as well as business owners. Nurses are required to have a knowledge base about disease processes and are expected to supply information when necessary to the physician to help improve the patient plan of care. Nurses are also more educated about the diseases that affect the patients for whom they care. Like the patients, nurses have access to peer reviewed data bases that give vast amounts of information on any specific subject they choose to research.

The role of a physician has also changed over the years. There are many women who are physicians, as well as physicians from other cultures. The training and education required to practice are much more intense than in the early years of the practice. Physicians have also developed their profession from what it was in the early years of medicine. They have developed specialized areas of practice, which require many years of study and training. The responsibility of deciding the course of treatment has usually fallen on the shoulders of the physician and this remains true today, for the most part.

Many physicians feel they have earned the right to have the last say in patient care, and they do have the higher level of education to make evidenced based judgments. While their role continues to be crucial, the fact is the final decision regarding the plan of care belongs, as it always has, to the patient; after all it is the patient's life that is affected by the outcomes of treatment. For years the patient has taken a passive role in his or her own plan of care, and until recently the physician did have the last say on what therapies to use, and the patient and the nurse just followed orders.

Because of these changes, the relationship dynamics between the three health care partners have to change into a more collaborative, respectful partnership in which everyone is working for a common goal of safe, effective patient care.

4. THE DYNAMICS OF THE THEORY OF MUTUAL RESPECT AND COLLABORATION

There are three dynamics in the theory: the patient-nurse, patient-physician, and nurse-physician relationships. Each of the dynamics has similar characteristics that need to be understood by everyone involved in creating and implementing an effective health care plan in order to cultivate mutual respect and collaboration. In this book the intention is to help the healthcare partners understand each other more and increase the collaboration between them. This process will help open communication and foster dynamics that will lead to improved outcomes for the patient and a better working climate for the nurse and physician. The authors also hope that the real life scenarios illustrating miscommunication and disrespect will help educate all the partners so they can avoid negative encounters with each other by reflecting on how these situations could have been handled differently. When any one of the partners, before reacting to someone's actions, takes a moment to pause and ask, "What is my reaction going to accomplish? Will I promote negativity and conflict, or can I help foster a caring and respectful dynamic?" communication generally improves. Respect is an essential element of all three dynamics involving the patient, nurse, and physician. Each of the healthcare partners must consider the others as valuable contributors who have unique knowledge, experience, and insight. Collaboration is not about who is in charge; it is working together to reach the common goal of improving a patient's healthcare status.

This theory has been developed because each of the health care dynamics often suffers from errors and miscommunication due to lack of respect and poor collaboration between the health care partners that create each dynamic. The lack of respect that some patients, nurses, and physicians show toward each other can hinder the collaboration needed to create and carry out an optimal plan of care. There is an existing problem with the way each of the dynamics perceives the other. Traditionally the roles were clear, but the roles of the patient and nurse have changed dramatically over the last 20 years. With this change, the way nurses and physicians view each other and the way they view the patient must change as well. This theory can be used by anyone, not just healthcare professionals. If all people attempted to treat others with the same respect and courtesy they want to receive, then effective communication would be much easier to achieve. In healthcare it is essential to be respectful of others when collaborating with them. Some patients may have many physicians at one time, each specializing in a different area of medicine. If each physician did not accept information from the other or from the nurse or patient, then the plan of care could be negatively affected, and chaos as to what orders to follow would arise. The traditional way the patient, nurse, and physician have functioned is no longer able to work in today's healthcare. A way to effectively collaborate and respect each other has to be developed and utilized by the practitioners in order to be productive.

As the three dynamics are discussed, real scenarios will be used to illustrate flaws in each dynamic. These scenarios have been submitted anonymously by individuals who wanted to share their stories. The names have been left out to protect the identity of the parties involved.

THE PATIENT AS KEY FACTOR IN HEALTH CARE DYNAMICS

When patients come to the hospital, it is because their health status has become unmanageable for the patients by themselves. For this reason they look to healthcare providers to make them well again or help return them to their previous state of health.

The patient is an individual, with unique expectations of what healthcare should be. Each patient has factors that make him or her unique. Such factors as culture, religion, socio-economic status, past experience, physical and mental abilities, and level of knowledge make the patient an influential partner in the plan of care. Since there is much diversity in the United States and the healthcare community, it is imperative for the healthcare providers to acknowledge these varied patient characteristics and work to ensure effective communication and collaboration with the patient to promote a strong, positive dynamic. Nurses and physicians must seek out this information from the patient and respect the patient's wishes when developing a plan of care.

The knowledge base of patients can vary widely. With technology today many patients have built a strong understanding about their diseases and health conditions. This can sometimes intimidate nurses and physicians when a patient appears to have as much knowledge or possibly even more than the healthcare provider. Progress may also be hindered when the patient's knowledge is based on unreliable sources and disputes the contributions made by the healthcare providers. Likewise when a patient does not have a strong knowledge base of his or her health conditions, the healthcare providers need to speak to the patient in terms the patient can understand, and not talk to the patient as though talking to a colleague.

Another consideration is the patient's ability to make his or her needs known. A patient may not be able make his or her needs known due to such variables as age, physical or mental ability, native language, or state of health. This scenario is usually handled by discussing the plan of care with the patient's next of kin, which can be a dilemma within itself because often family members do not agree on what should or should not be done. There have been many situations that have had to be settled by the court systems.

The patient's acceptance of the plan of care and his or her role as an active participant is also vital to the Theory of Mutual Respect and Collaboration. When a patient is non-compliant in the plan of care, the healthcare providers lose confidence in the patient and lose respect for the patient's contributions. When a patient is actively trying to improve his or her health, then healthcare providers are more eager to help. Many patients complain that the nurses and doctors do not care about them, and this is why they are non-compliant. A caring attitude cannot be conveyed without demonstration of respect. Many non-verbal actions can influence the cooperation of patients. If a patient feels staff members are being judgmental, this can hinder the implementation of the plan of care. Many patients look at the nurse's and physician's mannerisms, gestures, facial expressions, and tone of voice as cues to how the staff perceives them. It is very important for nurses and physicians to remain professional in the treatment of patients, so that the patient does not perceive a feeling of indifference. Therefore, nurses and physicians must not show personal biases to the patient.

Sometimes nurses and physicians are required to care for patients they may not like either personally or socially. This is when it is important for healthcare providers to maintain professionalism and provide care based on the patient's needs and not on the caregiver's biases. For example, patients and health care providers may have different beliefs regarding the use of blood products. The doctor may want to order a blood transfusion, but the patient may refuse that treatment. Once the healthcare provider has given the patient the risks and benefits of receiving blood products, the decision to not receive the product is up to the patient. Even if the healthcare providers think that it is essential for the health of the patient, they should refrain from trying to influence the patient's decision because of their beliefs.

In the traditional healthcare matrix, the physician makes the decisions and issues the orders, the nurse provides care and relays the orders to the patient, and the good patient does what the nurse and physician say. In this approach, the nurse conveys information from the patient to the physician, and then from the physician to the patient. This is where the breakdown in communication can start. Sometimes the nurse disregards the patient's information as not important and therefore does not report it to the doctor, or the information is given to the doctor who in turn disregards it as invalid. This may be due to a bias on the part of the nurse or doctor who may know the patient lacks an extensive medical knowledge base, and therefore considers the patient's information unimportant.

With modern technology and media readily available patients are increasingly more knowledgeable about healthcare and their own disease process, and they can be active participants in the development of their health care plans. Many patients have an in-depth knowledge of their own health and reactions to specific medicines or procedures through personal experience or research via the internet. The information they provide must be considered as pertinent by the healthcare team. This bias has slowly come to light as many healthcare providers have been patients themselves and seen firsthand how it feels to be a patient.

Surgery From _____ !!!

"As a nurse, I have not had many opportunities to be in the position of a patient or family member of a patient. So when I had surgery, it was a real eye opener for me to be in the role of a patient.

My experience started with having to be stuck six times before IV access could be established. This was very painful, but I did not complain because I knew it had to be done. Then I went to surgery, and as I was being wheeled down the hall, I became aware of just how scary it is to be the one being put to sleep. As a nurse I frequently take care of surgery patients, and it is routine for nurses to send patients to surgery and receive them back, but when I was the patient, it was not routine at all. I started thinking of all the things that can go wrong in surgery, such as a reaction to the anesthesia, a stroke, or myocardial infarction. So I was very scared for my family should something happen to me. It occurred to me how scary this must be for patients who have no medical knowledge, and realized that maybe nurses need to be more empathetic when taking care of patients who are going to surgery and not dismiss their concerns.

I did have my surgery and was very thankful that it had gone well, but as soon as I woke up, I realized my front teeth were broken. When I was intubated for the procedure, the anesthesiologist broke two of my front teeth; what was worse was they had left the broken teeth in my mouth. One tooth was flopping back and forth, so I took it out. This was concerning to me because I could have aspirated the tooth and had severe complications due to that.

In my next experience of being a patient, the nurses taking care of me did not know I was a nurse, so they treated me the way they would treat any other patient with no presumed medical knowledge, which is a scary thought. Through the night my IV infiltrated, and it woke me up because it was burning terribly. I called for the nurse to come and check my IV site. After about 30 minutes no one had come to check my IV, so I turned the pump off myself. Since I am a nurse, I considered that my nurse might be busy with a patient much sicker than I was. About one and a half hours later I pushed my call light again and was told someone would be in to check it because my nurse was on break. After another 30 minutes had passed another nurse came in and looked at my IV and said it was fine. I informed her about how badly it was burning and asked if she could please start another IV. The nurse clearly showed her frustration with my request. While this nurse was preparing to start a new IV site, my nurse finally came to my room and asked the other nurse what she was doing. She told my nurse that she was starting a new IV because I wanted one, and that my other IV site was fine. This was insulting to me because it was 1 o'clock in the morning, and if my IV site had been fine, I would have been happy to leave it in. I did not say anything to either nurse because I did not want to appear fussy even though I felt they were being rude to me.

The next thing that happened was my nurse came in about four hours later and took out my urinary catheter. I was very sleepy, but I told the nurse that I had packing that needed to be removed; she pulled back my blanket and stated, "No, you don't". Again I did not say anything, so when the day shift nurse came in about six hours after that and told me I needed to get up and use the restroom, I tried to tell her I had packing that needed to be removed. Yet again, this nurse did the same thing as the other nurse; she looked at me and said, "No, you don't". She then told me to get myself up and walk to the restroom. She did not try to help me get up out of bed or offer any kind of assistance. Luckily my husband was there, and he helped me get out of bed. I had an abdominal surgery and my incision was from hip to hip, so I was in a lot of pain. I made it to the restroom without any help from the nurse, but I still could not urinate. I sat back down on the side of the bed and being very frustrated at this point, I told the nurse to go call my doctor and ask her about the packing. This nurse left the room and came back a few minutes later with my doctor's assistant, and said to him, "She says she has packing, but she doesn't." The physician assistant then informed the nurse that I did in fact have packing, and she proceeded to remove the packing with the nurse in the room. I was then able to urinate.

This whole ordeal was very educational for me because it showed me that nurses do not always value the information that patients give them, and this is a very big error on the nurse's part. What if I had been someone with no medical knowledge and did not question the nurses? If I had been sent home with that packing, I could have developed severe complications such as an infection or even sepsis."   -Anonymous Nurse/Patient

In this scenario there was breakdown in communication between the nurses and the patient because of the nurses' bias that they had more knowledge than the patient. This situation resulted in creating distrust and resentment instead of promoting mutual respect. The behaviors of the nursing staff did not put the patient at ease with the competency of healthcare being provided. The collaboration between the nurses and the patient was hindered because of the unwillingness of the nurses to accept the patient's information as valid. As a result the patient became frustrated and resentful, was made to feel uncomfortable, and was put in danger of developing severe complications.

This is why it is important for medical staff and healthcare providers to respect the patient's information as valid and investigate his or her concerns. In the Theory of Mutual Respect and Collaboration the nurses would have avoided these problems by viewing the patient as an individual with knowledge of her illness or injury, the ability to express needs and concerns, and an awareness of what each healthcare provider had already done or communicated. This would have led the nurse to accept the patient's information as valid and to address the patient's concerns. If this theory had been applied, mutual respect between the nurses and the patient would have been established and the collaboration between the two could have been more effective. The patient would have been more relaxed going into surgery, would not have been left for over two hours without the medicine or fluids that the IV was providing, and would never have been at risk of being sent home with the surgery packing still in place.

Neo-Natal Nurse Nightmare

"I was a young mother whose baby was born prematurely and hospitalized for six weeks. The experience was terrifying. I was not allowed to see my baby because she was so sick and premature. One of the nurses went above and beyond the call of duty. That nurse took pictures of my baby while she was in the NICU on her camera phone and would come out and show me. This meant so much to me because I could not hold her, but at least I could see pictures of her. When my baby was finally moved to a room where I could hold her, there was a nurse there who was terrible. I would go up to the nurse's desk to request things such as more formula or diapers, and the nurse would be on a social media website and ignore me. I would say, "Excuse me," after a few minutes, and then she would acknowledge that I was there. She would show her frustration when she would have to get up and get the things that I needed to take care of my baby. I even heard her use obscene language as she would get up sometimes. I came close to reporting her, but I was afraid that the times I was not there she would be mean to my baby. So I never said anything about it, but I do not recommend that hospital to anyone because of that one nurse."   -*Anonymous mother of a neo-natal patient*

In this scenario even though there was one nurse whom the young mother liked, the dislike for the other nurse far outweighed the positive relationship and created a negative perception of that hospital. The nurse that displayed such poor professionalism did not foster mutual respect for this patient and the family. The effort to communicate and collaborate on the young mother's behalf was met with a negative reception by the nurse. When the nurse displayed such a negative attitude and lack of compassion, the young mother could not accept the nurse as someone who valued patients, and trust was broken, not only between the mother and the nurse, but between the mother and the entire hospital. When a patient or the patient's family does not trust the nurses or doctors who are caring for them, then the plan of care cannot proceed effectively. In this case the mother could have been intimidated to the point of not properly taking care of the young infant.

Control Freak Nurses

"Recently my mother had to be placed in a nursing home because her dementia had become worse, and it was not safe to leave her by herself. Needless to say, I felt terrible about having to place her in the nursing home, and I had a tremendous amount of guilt. My mother had fallen and required surgery prior to being placed in the nursing home. Her doctor told us that she would have a lot of pain. So the one thing I felt I could do was to make sure that my mother was not in excruciating pain all the time. When I would visit my mother, she would hold her knee and complain about how badly it hurt. I knew she had pain medicine ordered, so I would ask her nurse to give her pain medicine. The nurse would say, "If I give her something now, then she won't get any medicine tonight." I knew that my mother was supposed to get her pain medicine twice a day, and every eight hours as needed for breakthrough pain. The nurse would then offer acetaminophen. I did not want to argue with the nurse, so I did not say anything. About a week later when I went to see my mother, she was hurting again, and I again asked her nurse if she could have acetaminophen. This same nurse said, "Well if I give her acetaminophen now then, she can't have her pain medicine tonight." I asked her why not. She said it would be too much acetaminophen. At this point I became very angry, but I still did not say anything because I could tell the nurse would have been argumentative about anything.

I am still considering going to the director of the facility to report that particular nurse because she did not consider my mother's pain in her effort to create a power struggle between me and her. I do not like complaining about staff, but this nurse should have been concerned with my mother and not trying to show me who was boss."   -Disgruntled Daughter

In this scenario the nurse's decision to not give the pain medicine created tension between the patient's daughter and herself. Many nurses confuse a family member's request with a demand, and then they try to control the situation by refusing to give medicine or perform some other task that normally they would do happily. As was stated by the family member this situation should have been about the patient and not the nurse and the family member. The nurse should have reflected on the situation and considered that the patient did have orders for pain medicine and was requesting it. Instead of treating the patient, the nurse's actions led to the daughter harboring harsh feelings toward her, and very possibly the entire nursing home. Fortunately the daughter did not retaliate, as might have happened in some cases.

Nurses need to consider the request of the patient and family member as valid, and not try to manipulate the orders to exert their authority. When this happens, it creates disrespect between those that should be partners and impedes the effectiveness of the plan of care. Some other negative results included the patient not getting the pain medicine she needed, which could have led her to react negatively, not eat properly, or not exercise the joint. The daughter was left with a conflict between what the doctor had ordered and said was permissible with what the nurse said was allowable; this could create doubt about future treatment the doctor might order. Also if the doctor found out that the nurse had been circumventing his/her orders, that would have led the doctor to distrust the nurse in other matters.

In the Theory of Mutual Respect and Collaboration there are many ways that effective communication can be achieved. One of the most important ways is to acknowledge a patient and his or her family members. When a patient or family member comes to the nurse's station, the nurse should acknowledge that person. When a person feels ignored, this sends a clear message that he or she is not considered important. This can lead to many negative emotions for the patient and/or family members. It is crucial to building a trusting relationship among all the partners that patient, nurse, and physician acknowledge and truly listen to each other. The patient's information is the basis of the plan of care, so why would nurses and physicians want to ignore what they have to say? Paying attention early on can save much time and effort later; it may even save a life.

It is a common fact that some patients can be a little on the theatrical side or even outright unbelievable with their contribution of information. Many patients have complaints of chronic pain that never seems to get relieved with medicine. Some are more vocal with their complaints than others. This is when nurses and physicians may lose respect for the patient's information. When this happens, it creates a divide in the patient-nurse-doctor relationship dynamics. As healthcare professionals the nurses and physicians should put aside personal biases no matter what the scenario is, treat all patients with respect, and value their contribution to the plan of care. Healthcare providers are not to pass judgment, but rather provide service to patients. This includes the patients that are not particularly likable to a nurse or physician. When a patient feels that he or she is not being taken seriously, this creates animosity. Healthcare providers should remain professional and reassure the patient that complaints are being taken seriously, and they will try to help the patient achieve a resolution appropriate to his or her health concerns.

It may be that the patient's information or concerns are truly invalid. This would require a slightly different approach. The care provider should first seriously consider the patient's information, but if it is untrustworthy or inaccurate, the provider should acknowledge that the patient has concerns– just maybe not the ones being voiced. This would mean treating the patient with respect (as the provider may not know why the patient is not reliable), but also with extra caution.

A common mistake made by healthcare professionals is to stereotype patients. When this happens, a barrier to communication is quickly established. It is difficult to communicate with patients who are already resentful of nurses and physicians from previous encounters. In these situations nurses and physicians need to take an opportunity to reassure such patients that judgment is not being made on them, and that their complaints are being taken seriously. Most patients will modify their behavior if they feel they are being respected by the staff. For harmonious patient-nurse-physician relationships, it is imperative that the healthcare providers treat each patient with respect and dignity, no matter how they view the patient personally. Health care providers have a job to serve patients, and to do so professionally and with an open mind; they do not have to agree with the patient's lifestyle or beliefs, but they do need to respect the patient and not show their own personal biases. This approach will help ensure open communication and a more effective plan of care.

Not So Nice Nurses

"My daughter was 12 years old when she developed epilepsy. She had always been my healthy child; she very rarely got sick. She was at school one day, and the school nurse called and told me that I needed to get to the school right away. An ambulance had been called; apparently my daughter had a seizure at school.

I rode in the ambulance with my daughter to the hospital. When we arrived in the emergency room, the nurses were very busy attending to patients. The ambulance team left my daughter in a hall on a stretcher, and I was standing beside her and holding her hand. She was in some sort of drowsy state and did not know what had happed.

A nurse came up to her and started asking me questions, like, "What happened?" I told her that I was not sure because I was not there when it happened. She then proceeded to ask me if my daughter was on drugs and alcohol. I told her no; she said in a very accusing tone, "Are you sure?" To which I replied, "Yes, I am." I was very scared about what had happened with my daughter, and I wanted to find out why she had a seizure, but this nurse seemed very rude to me. The nurse then smacked my hand lightly, the one I was using to hold my daughter's hand. She said, "Move; I need to assess her." I was already upset over my daughter being sick, and this nurse's rude behavior just about pushed me over the edge. I refrained from saying anything to her for fear that my daughter would be mistreated.

They did admit my daughter to the hospital, and the staff members on the floor where she was placed were equally rude. They acted as if my daughter was faking it. It was not until my daughter had a seizure in front of them, and her drug screen had come back negative and the EEG showed epileptic form discharges that the nurses and doctors started treating my daughter like she was really sick. I know that nurses and doctors may see a lot of fakers in their line of work, but they should not think everyone is faking it. Whatever happened to innocent until proven guilty? Nurses and doctors should take a patient's complaint of illness seriously until tests prove otherwise."

-Distraught Mother

Sometimes in healthcare nurses and physicians do tend to stereotype patients, but it is very important not to form preconceived judgments of patients. In the scenario above the patient did have a legitimate health problem. The cold and judgmental behavior of the nurses made a difficult and scary time for the mother of the patient even worse. When nurses and doctors give the impression that a patient is not really sick, this causes a barrier to form and communication is hindered. Once the barrier is up, it is hard to break it down. The patients and their families no longer trust the opinions of the medical personnel. This is especially true when the patient proves the first judgments of doctors and nurses were wrong. When this occurs, many patients or their families request a transfer to another facility.

In the current healthcare market there is a lot of competition for patients. There are many hospitals closing their doors because of decreased patient loads. Patients are willing to travel longer distances to receive quality health care. This makes it especially important that health care providers treat patients with respect and dignity. Even if they may think the patient is 'faking it,' they should never let that show. In the scenario above the nurse should have shown more compassion for the patient's mother, instead of the rude behavior she exhibited. Showing more empathy simply by keeping her suspicions to herself would have garnered more respect toward the staff. Instead the patient's mother did not trust the staff. In today's healthcare market this kind of behavior from nurses and doctors can have a large monetary effect on a hospital if the patients demand to be transferred to a place where they are treated better.

Dr. Mean and Hateful

"When I had my first pregnancy, I was assigned a doctor by the clinic that I went to. This doctor was old and not very nice at all. He was very rough when he did exams on me, to the point I would leave in tears. As my abdomen grew from being pregnant, he would measure my stomach. He had a long thumb nail; all the rest of his finger nails were trimmed except the one thumb nail. He would press the thumb nail into my side to hold the measuring tape. When I told him that that hurt, he replied, "It is going to hurt a lot worse than that before it is over with." (He was referring to the pain of giving birth). I had three office visits with him and each one was humiliating, painful or both. On the last visit I had with him I asked him how far along I was in my pregnancy. He looked at me over top of his glasses and said, "The only ones who can tell that are the ones who were there that night." I was so offended at his comments that when I left the exam room to go to the checkout window, I told the receptionist that if I had to have him as a doctor, I would just as soon have my baby at home. Fortunately for me there was another doctor at the clinic. I started seeing him, and he was a great doctor with a great personality. I think the other doctor retired not long after that, and he really needed to because he acted like he hated his job and his patients." -*Mother to Be*

In this scenario the physician treated the patient with disrespect, and this ended up costing him the patient. Whether or not he hated his practice, was just tired, or did not like the patient is irrelevant. The physician had an obligation to provide quality health care to the patient and did not. Many health care providers do not consider having a good bedside manner as part of giving quality health care, but patients have the right to choose whom they want to provide their health care. Having a good bedside manner is essential for patient satisfaction. Physicians and nurses need to respect the patient and offer empathy to them.

Another reason this is important is that in the recent health care reform Medicare is planning reimbursment based on patient satisfaction scores. This means physicians and nurses need to ensure that they are doing what they can to make the patients feel at ease and comforatble with the care they are receiving. Hospitals and health care facilities with poor patient satisfaction scores will receive less reimbursement. Hospitals with high patient satisafaction scores will receive bonuses. ("Medicare To Begin Basing Hospital Payments On Patient-Satisfaction Scores", 2011) The bottom line is when pateints are not happy with the care provided, providers and hospitals could be seeing it reflected on their financial statements.

Treated Like A Criminal

"My husband had been trying to taper himself off an antianxiety medication, with the approval of his psychiatrist. The problem was that about halfway through the process, he became very anxious and depressed. His psychiatrist was not in the office, so he suggested that I take my husband to the emergency room so that he could get some medications to act quickly to help resolve his anxiety and depression. This seemed logical to me, so I took my husband to the emergency room expecting help; what we received was entirely different.

When my husband and I were taken to the exam room, the nurse asked what had brought him in. My husband tried to explain to her that he had been trying to taper off a medication by himself and had come to a point that his anxiety and depression had gotten out of control. The nurse just looked at him and turned away. As she was turning, she rolled her eyes in very rudely. She went to the door and yelled, "I need a security guard in here!" I did not know why she would think that she needed security because my husband was not being hostile or rude in any way. Then the doctor came in and started asking my husband questions like, " Have you ever thought of killing yourself?" My husband said "No," but he did mention to the doctor that ten years earlier when he was 18 years old, he was arguing with his mother and had said, "I wish I was dead", and his mother took him to a psych center. He also told the doctor that he was only joking back then, but his mother thought he was serious. The doctor then left the room.

The next thing we knew my husband was placed under a 72 hour hold and could not leave. I questioned the doctors, but all they would say is that he had suicidal thoughts. I tried to explain that he had made a comment to his mother ten years ago, but that he was not suicidal now. They would not listen to me; I felt helpless because there was nothing I could do or say that would convince them my husband just needed a little medication to help him because the prescribed medicine he was on had already gotten out of his system, and it would take two weeks to build up the levels again, and that was why we came to the ER and why the psychiatrist suggested we come in the first place.

All this fell on deaf ears. I felt as though the doctor and nurses did not even listen to us; they just made asumptions and stereotyped my husband as someone who was on severe drugs, and then treated us without regard for what was really wrong with him. To make matters worse, we were held in the ER for five hours, and around one am the police arrived and shackled my husband's hands and feet to lead him out of the emergency room. I still have no idea why they treated us this way. My husband had not made any threats to anyone, and he was not exhibiting any violent behavior whatsoever. I was humiliated and embarrassed for my husband and myself. My husband works and pays his taxes, and he was treated like some sort of hardened criminal. I was devastated.

Then we were taken to a mental health clinic to wait until my husband could be taken to a psych center. While we were there, a nurse came by the room and said out loud, " It's a full moon; looks like all the crazies are out." I was very angry at the way my husband and I were treated by these so called professionals, when there was nothing professional about them at all. At the suggetion of my husband's psychiatrist we went to the emergency room for help to get my husband some fast acting anti-anxiety medicine; what we endured was disrespect and four days of pure hell. This should never have happened to us. If the nurses and doctors would have listened to us and not made assumptions, it would not have. "

 - *Frustrated wife with husband being stereo-typed*

In this scenario the nurses and physicians made judgements about the patient's condition. The patient was subjected to a horrible ordeal that was unneccesary. If the nurses and physicians had been willing to listen to the patient and his wife, they would have realized that the patient had just reached a low level on his medication and needed a temporary boost until the patient was able to see his psychiatrist in the office. This scenario could have been handled differently if the physician had listened to the patient; instead the patient's reason for being there was dismissed most likely due to assumptions made by the physician regarding his mental state. They did not try to contact the patient's psychiatrist, did not give any credence to the wife's explanations, and made very unprofessional casual comments that should never have been uttered. The patient and his wife suffered public humiliation as a result of some very closed minded health care providers.

THE NURSE AS KEY FACTOR IN HEALTH CARE DYNAMICS

Nursing has been defined in many ways over the years. In the early years of the nursing profession, nurses were expected to be subservient to the physicians. They were never to question any decisions made by the physicians. Some people still have this view. Today nurses have much more responsibility than in previous eras. Nurses are now required to be more knowledgeable about diseases and disease processes and are held accountable for their own errors, such as giving the wrong medication, as well as their inactions concerning doctors who prescribe the wrong treatment or medicine. This new level of responsibility requires a new view of the nurse's role as a partner in providing health care. The definition of nursing by today's standards is: a partner who provides both health care and education to promote healthy lifestyles and who serves as a patient advocate. All this makes the nurse a critical and dynamic contributor to the plan of care. Nurses must be familiar with each patient's health status indicators such as lab values, diagnostic reports, medications, and general patient status as reported by the patient, family, and nurses or aides. The nurse reports this information to the physician, and then serves as a collaborative partner in improving the patient's health status.

While patients and physicians both have much greater expectations of nurses and demand that nurses have much more knowledge, skill, and education, many nurses still feel that they are not given the respect they have earned and deserve. This feeling of not being respected can lead to failed communication which has a very negative effect on all three of the health care dynamics. This is the purpose of the Theory of Mutual Respect and Collaboration-- to eliminate the assumptions that can lead to disrespect, poor communication, and ineffective collaboration and to open new ways to build respect and successful collaboration so that all three health care dynamics function optimally ensuring a patient receives the best care possible.

The nurse is an individual and a healthcare provider. As individuals nurses have their own beliefs, experiences, and cultural influences that affect their perceptions of the plan of care. Many nurses do not even realize they have a bias when it comes to the other partners on the health care team. Many nurses have stated that they stereotyped patients, especially those who come in with complaints of chronic pain. They may not even realize they have a bias toward patients with complaints of pain, but they do not take the patients' complaints seriously and the patients may become very aware of the bias. This can lead to the patient feeling disrespected, which can lead to a breakdown in communication within the healthcare team.

The nurse's knowledge base is also a factor in the health care dynamics involving nursing. Some nurses have a broader knowledge base than others. It is important to consider the level of experience the nurse has, as well as the knowledge retained from formal education and training. Some nurses have a better ability to retain information than others. Nurses who do not retain information easily may feel intimidated by patients, doctors or even other nurses when their decisions or actions are questioned. It is important for patients and physicians to consider the experience level of a nurse when discussing the plan of care with them.

The ability of the nurse also plays a role in the way the other health care partners view him or her, so it is important for nurses to conduct themselves in a professional manner. When a nurse does not possess the skills necessary to maintain the level of expertise expected of nurses today, a breakdown in the communication is likely. Also important in the Theory of Mutual Respect and Collaboration is the nurse's ability to convey the needed information correctly between the other health care partners. While the nurse expects his or her contributions to be accepted or at least respected during the development of a healthcare plan, the nurse must also be careful to show respect for the contributions of both physician and patient. Having a caring attitude toward the patient as well as the physician is also conducive to mutual respect. Many nurses feel they do not have the respect of the patients or the physicians, so they in turn do not display a caring attitude. This behavior just leads to distrust. Doctors and patients also have their strengths and weaknesses. The nurse must be able to respectfully provide assistance in helping to improve their problem areas. If done in the right manner, such guidance will usually be welcomed or at least appreciated. Keeping quiet or criticizing in the wrong manner, may lead to conflict or, even worse, result in harm to a patient.

Dr. Know it all/ Not so much

"I was taking care of a patient who had a femoral bypass surgery and was scheduled to go home that day. The patient had been on an IV drip, and it was down to 2mcg. On the orders of the patient's primary physician I gave the patient 36mg of the same medication by mouth, waited 2 hours and turned the drip off. About 3 hours later the patient started having frequent PVC's, so I called the cardiologist on the patient's case to inform him of the situation. While I was on hold waiting for the doctor, the patient's rhythm changed and when the doctor came to the phone, I informed him of the changed rhythm, and I stated that I thought he was having a MI. The doctor asked me if I was a doctor. I told him, "No, I am not a doctor, but I have seen enough heart attacks to know what one looks like." The doctor proceeded to inform me the patient was not having a heart attack; it was because I had turned off the IV drip abruptly. We disagreed for about five minutes; meanwhile, the patient was getting into serious trouble, so I asked one of the nurses there to get the heart surgeon on the phone so I could get help for this patient. Luckily for me and the patient the surgeon was in the unit and came to us quickly. While I was still on the phone with the cardiologist and being insulted by him, the surgeon walked in and looked at the patient's rhythm and stated, "This patient is having a heart attack." I handed the surgeon the phone, and said, "Tell that to Dr. ...., because he won't listen to me; I am just a nurse."

The surgeon convinced the cardiologist of the urgency of the situation, and the patient was taken to the cath lab. He came back on a balloon pump because one of his coronary arteries was 99% occluded. I was so frustrated at the disrespect shown to me by this doctor that I have not had much respect for him since. I felt I did what I had to do for my patient, but I felt helpless until the surgeon came in and made the cardiologist understand how serious the patient's condition was. I felt like my experience as a critical care nurse did not mean anything. "

-Anonymous Critical Care Nurse

In this scenario the nurse was attempting to have an open dialogue with the physician about a patient's condition. The physician did not respect the nurse's assessment of the situation. This disrespect led to the nurse distrusting the physician's ability to make appropriate decisions in critical situations. In this situation there was a proper resolution made to the patient's condition, but this is not always the case. Some physicians do not accept the nurse's ability to interpret data appropriately, and this leads to barriers in communication.

This has been a problem in the nurse – physician dynamic for years. One of the problems is that it has been a tradition that the nurse be subservient to the physician and not question or have an opinion about the plan of care. Nurses have traditionally been expected to follow doctor's orders, but now with healthcare changing, this expectation is also changing. Nurses are now required to have higher levels of formal education and are expected to know how to take care of patients in rapidly changing situations. The higher level of training means that more is expected of nurses today than ever before. Nurses are with the patient more than the physicians are and they can tell when the patient's condition has changed.

Nurses are also being held accountable for their actions or inactions when it comes to patient safety. For this reason, a climate of mutual respect between nurse and physician has to be established in order to have effective communication and collaboration. There have been some lawsuits of malpractice against physicians and the nurses in the case are being sued as well because the courts are saying that the nurses have the level of expertise needed to know if the physician is practicing in an unsafe manner or doing a procedure unnecessarily. This is where the culture of the roles of the nurse--physician relationship has to change. Since nurses are being held accountable for patients in their care, they are attempting to have a more active role in the plan of care for the patient. Sometimes physicians can be disrespectful to nurses for unknown reasons; maybe they are tired, overworked, or having personal issues. Nonetheless, this disrespect can lead to feelings of inadequacy for the nurse.

While the nurse expects his or her contributions to be accepted or at least respected during the development of a healthcare plan, the nurse must also be careful to show respect for the contributions of both physician and patient. Having a caring attitude toward the patient as well as the physician is very conducive to mutual respect. Many nurses feel they do not have the respect of the patients or the physicians, so they in turn do not display a caring attitude. This behavior just creates more distrustful dynamics.

Dr. Stuck In The Past

"I remember one morning several years ago, there was an older doctor who had very old school opinions of what the nurse's role should be. After I had reviewed my patient's labs, that doctor came in. I approached him to inform him about the abnormal labs. I got as far as, "I was going to let you know this patient's potassium level was..," and he put his hand up in my face as if to tell me to shut up, and proceeded to tell me that lab values were not my business; they were his. He then went on to tell me I should stick to bed pans and bed baths as that was my job. Luckily for me there was a flyer hanging on the wall of the nursing station that stated that nurses were to report all abnormal labs to the doctors. I pointed to the flyer and told him that reporting the labs to him was my job, and he could do whatever he wanted with the information." -*Anonymous Nurse*

In this scenario the physician had preconceived notions about the nurse's role. Such limited views of the role of nurses are still held by many physicians today, and need to change because nurses are responsible for much more than bed pans and bed baths. Nurses are patient advocates; in order to communicate effectively with doctors they have to know much more about patients than they did in bygone eras. Nurses have to know each patient's history, medications, and plan of care, and they must update each consulting physician about the other physicians' plans so information is not missed. Nurses have to know whether the patient is going to have surgery or any other procedures that require the patient to not eat; also it is the nurse's responsibility to make sure the patient does not eat or drink and takes the appropriate pre – medicines for any scheduled procedures. Nurses have to have this knowledge about every patient that is in their care that day. It is also nurses' responsibility to complete all required documentation for all of their patients. This includes all the admission and discharges that come through. Given the scope of all the responsibility nurses have on a daily basis and the knowledge base that is required of them in today's healthcare arena, nurses should be considered one of the key contributors in the plan of care. Over the years many nurses have challenged the traditional treatment of nurses and have helped shape the role of nurses today. Many physicians do consider nurses as a vital component to the plan of care, but there are still many physicians who have an antiquated view of nurses as being subservient to them. This is the culture that must change. The way physicians view and treat nurses is crucial to the progression of modern medicine and the collaboration needed for providing excellent healthcare service.

Dr. Real Jerk

"I witnessed a physician being very disrespectful to a nurse who did not have a lot of experience. It was about five pm and the physician had been consulted to put in a central venous line because peripheral IVs could not be established. The physician came in and asked why the nurse waited so late in the day to get the consult. The nurse tried to explain that many nurses had tried to get peripheral access and were unsuccessful, but he did not let her finish what she was saying. He put his hand up in a motion to shut her up and said, "You are an incompetent nurse." The nurse's face went completely red. This doctor very arrogantly embarrassed and humiliated her. Needless to say she was very flustered after that, and she was on the verge of crying the whole time the doctor was there. I just thought it was exceptionally rude for the doctor to treat her that way, and it was totally unnecessary."

-*Anonymous nurse*

In this scenario the physician allowed his personal bias to get in the way of effective communication with the nurse. This behavior of doctors speaking to nurses in a disrespectful manner and the culture that allows it should not be accepted in the healthcare industry today. No matter what the personal problems, views, or biases are of one person, doctors should treat people they work with and care for with respect. In the Theory of Mutual Respect the physician respects the nurse's contribution to the plan of care and demonstrates the same respect he or she expects. Such behavior can have several negative effects. The nurse may simply choose to not interact with the doctor, meaning that the doctor will most likely not get all of the information he might need to make good decisions. In the above the scenarios, the nurse was "on the verge of crying", a condition that is likely to have a negative impact on her ability to perform her duties. If a patient witnesses such an act, the patient may also be intimidated and withhold information or decide that the doctor did not care about others.

Nurses not only need the respect of the physicians, they also need the respect of the patient. Healthcare has trended toward patient satisfaction and making sure the patient's needs are met. There is not much data on how the patient should behave toward the nurse and physician. Just as many patients have experienced rude and obnoxious behavior from healthcare employees, so have the healthcare employees had to endure disrespect from patients. Of course, it is the job of the healthcare employees to always act professionally, and treating a disrespectful patient with disrespect does nothing to improve the situation and usually makes matters much worse. However, patients should also understand how they may only be hurting themselves when they choose to behave rudely.

Pain in The ____ Patient

"One of the rudest patients I have ever had to care for was a man who came in for chest pain. All of his lab work and diagnostic tests were normal, but he insisted he was having chest pain and the only thing that helped it was morphine. He did not want nitro, just the morphine. He called me to his room to complain that he needed more pain meds, and insisted that I was going to have to call the doctor to get more. He also complained that he had not received the extra sandwich he had ordered from the cafeteria. I apologized to him that he had to wait and told him that I would call the cafeteria for him; and then I asked him if there was anything else I could do. He used some obscene language and said, "Yeah go get me a soda." I went to the nutrition room and brought the patient a soda; I asked him if there was anything else I could do for him, and he said "Yeah, now go get me some ice." I could see that he was being derogatory, so I said, "Okay, tell me everything you want so I can get it all at one time." By this time his sandwich had been brought in, and he picked it up and threw it against the wall, and said, "I want a new nurse." I told him that I could make that happen.

I ran into a problem though; no other nurses working that day would take him as a patient because of the way he disrespected the staff. Unfortunately we have to put up with a lot of verbal abuse like this in the effort to keep patient satisfaction scores up. I wish patients had to show us some respect."   *-Anonymous nurse*

Many nurses express frustration that they do not get the respect from patients and doctors that they feel they deserve. Traditionally nurses were not supposed to show any concern for their own opinions in the work place, but nurses are crucial in the patient-nurse-physician healthcare dynamics. Respect from the patient and the physician is imperative for the nurse to feel as though his or her contributions are important. When patients disrespect the nurse's effort to help in the plan of care, the nurse is not inspired or motivated to have a caring attitude toward the patient. The whole encounter will then spiral further into a breakdown in communication.

Patients need to understand the importance of mutual respect between patients and the nurses and physicians caring for them in order to help build effective working relationships. The nurse and patient must agree to establish a trusting, respectful and collaborative relationship as soon as the patient seeks out healthcare whether at a medical office or hospital. Both must strive to respect the other no matter what their personal differences are. This will enable them to work together in an effective collaborative manner to create a trusting relationship. This agreement must be extended to the physician upon his or her arrival as well. Physicians and nurses have to set an example to the patient by respecting each other's contributions to the plan of care. Leading by example is the best way to educate patients about how to respect the other contributors to the plan of care.

It is very unprofessional for staff to argue and or be disrespectful to one another in front of the patient. When a patient is a witness to such a display by professionals, they are not inspired to show respect to either healthcare provider. Maintaining professionalism and being courteous to colleagues is crucial to obtaining the respect of the patient.

Noisy Nurses

"I was working one day and two nurses started arguing loudly in front of patients and visitors. The fuss occurred because one nurse felt she was working harder than the other. The nurse who was upset, walked up to the other nurse who was sitting at the desk and said, "It must be nice to be able to sit around while everyone else is working." The nurse who was sitting responded with, "I just sat down, and it is nice to get my job done and be able to sit down a few minutes." The conversation grew into a loud argument that clearly caused other co-workers, patients, and visitors to be uneasy. I just do not think that was the time or the place to do this. Staff should not argue in front of patients." -Anonymous Nurse

The stress of the job can overwhelm some staff, and many have reacted to a situation before thinking it through, as in this scenario. On both sides of the argument, the nurse who was upset first would have gained more respect if she would have approached the other nurse and asked for help if that nurse had the time. Also the nurse sitting should have tried to de-escalate the situation when she saw the frustration of the other nurse. Had both nurses had been willing to pause a second and reflect on how their actions could cause unfavorable reactions from each other, this scenario might have been avoided.

In a health care setting sometimes the stress of the job can be overwhelming and tempers can cause disputes between co-workers. It is imperative for nurses and physicians to maintain the professionalism they were taught in school and look for alternative methods to settle differences. One thing that should never happen is for staff to argue or disrespect each other in front of patients, visitors, or other staff members. When there are disputes, the parties involved should settle their arguments in private. This is the best policy to maintain the level of professionalism that is expected from healthcare providers.

The nurse to nurse relationship needs to be

examined also. It has been said that nurses often eat their young. Many seasoned nurses do not appreciate the contributions of new nurses and do not readily accept any information a new nurse has on a plan of care. Even if the seasoned nurse thinks the information is correct, many times she or he does not express this to the new nurse. This dismissal of the new nurse's contribution can make the new nurse feel unimportant. Rather than promoting feelings of inadequacy, the seasoned nurse should foster a more collaborative work environment whereby the new nurse is not intimidated and is encouraged to share ideas. Likewise, new nurses do need to show respect for the experienced nurses who have been in practice and have a working knowledge of nursing. When a new nurse shows arrogance, this is not conducive to a collaborative work environment. Nurses from all levels of expertise can learn from each other. The new nurses are often up to date on many new technologies and healthcare innovations, and the seasoned nurses have pearls of wisdom and reality based experience from years of nursing. In the Theory of Mutual Respect colleagues work together for a common goal by sharing ideas and experience to improve the services offered by a health care team.

THE PHYSICIAN AS A KEY FACTOR IN HEALTHCARE DYNAMICS

The physician is an individual and a health care

provider. Each physician has a diverse background and is influenced by his or her culture, education, family, past experiences, and beliefs that make him or her unique. Trying to fit individual beliefs and cultural expectations into the plan of care for patients may be very difficult for some physicians. It is very hard for healthcare providers to put aside their own cultures and embrace the culture of others. While it not necessary to embrace the other culture, it is absolutely essential to respect and try to understand other cultures in order to develop an excellent plan of care for a patient. Healthcare providers must respect the cultures of their patients no matter how different those beliefs or practices are from their own, and they must incorporate the patient's wishes into the plan of care.

The physician's knowledge base is different from the other healthcare partners. All physicians go through extensive training and board exams in order to be licensed. Physicians also have to stay current in their knowledge by completing continuing education requirements and sitting for their boards every ten years. Some physicians go into specialty areas that require even more extensive training. As with any field there are some physicians who have practiced longer and are more experienced than others. There are also some young physicians who may lack years of experience but are extremely gifted in their knowledge of medicine.

The physician's ability to make decisions is

improved with extensive training and education, but no matter how well trained, a physician can still come across cases beyond his or her expertise. This is one reason there are many physicians in specialty areas. Many internal medicine physicians will consult specialists for areas that go beyond their training. This division of focus may lead to communication issues, especially when several physicians are caring for one patient and are not collaborating effectively with each other about the plan of care.

Physicians sometimes find it difficult to accept information from a nurse or patient. One reason for this is that physicians are responsible for developing a plan of care for a patient, and all physicians take this responsibility very seriously. Many physicians feel they are being asked to relinquish their authority by including input from the patient and the nurse, when in fact collaboration does not require the physician to leave the decision making to the patient and nurse. Another reason may be that some physicians have a bias that whatever knowledge the patient or nurse has is not as important as that of the physician. When physicians can get past their own biases toward the other contributors, they can work with them more effectively.

A caring attitude is something that all physicians possess to some extent. Physicians have been traditionally taught about caring for patients from birth to death. Each physician's caring attitude is demonstrated differently based on his or her own culture and beliefs. Some physicians put less emphasis on establishing mutual respect with patients than they do on establishing a caring relationship with them. Basically they feel "doctor knows best" and just want the patient to comply so he or she can be taken care of.

Another issue that may hinder the establishment of mutual respect is the differences in knowledge levels of physicians, nurses, and patients. Physicians have been perceived as highly respected and educated professionals in nearly every culture. All over the world getting accepted into medical school is very competitive. Furthermore, becoming a doctor is a very stressful and demanding process of reading and studying, taking tests and national exams, and completing clinical rotations and internships. Licensing is also very difficult in all parts of the world. Also most doctors have gone through further training, so it takes about ten to fifteen years to become a physician who can practice medicine independently. When a doctor graduates from medical school after such a long process, there is a mindset that they know it all.

Historically doctors have been perceived as the last word on patient care. Doctors still give orders, not requests. As doctors have gone through various physical, emotional, mental training and education, they have become better prepared than anyone else to take care of patients. Traditionally doctors have not been questioned by nurses and other caregivers, but now with the advent of the internet, knowledge is more accessible to nurses and patients. Most of the patients and nurses conduct internet based research about their own particular health problems or diseases before the doctor even evaluates them. The question is: can internet research be enough or equivalent to the ten to fifteen years of rigorous training it takes to become a doctor? Some of the nurses, patients, and caregivers may think that it is close enough. How to use the tools of this new era of smart phones and internet for better patient care and collaboration between doctors and nurses without letting available facts substitute for true education and wisdom is a fine line. On one side we have chaos, and on the other side collaboration.

Dr. Cut Throat

"I was taking care of a post- operative patient, and the surgeon had ordered IV antibiotics. The internal medicine doctor on the case said the patient did not need the antibiotics because the patient's white blood cell count was within normal limits. The surgeon came in later that day and was upset that the antibiotics were stopped. He asked me why I stopped the antibiotics, and I told him I didn't stop them, another doctor did. He asked me why I did not call him about it before I stopped the antibiotics. I told him I didn't think about it. He had a medical student with him and looked at her and said, "This is one of the problems; nurses think they know everything, but they don't know anything." The doctor looked at me and said, "Isn't that right?" I said, "I don't think I know everything," and I walked away. I was hurt and humiliated by the behavior of this doctor, and I have not liked him since. I will not try to help him anymore if he needs it."

-Anonymous Nurse

In this scenario the physician was very disrespectful to the nurse. Instead of insulting her, he should have discussed the cancelation of his orders with the physician that did it. This is another problem in the collaboration process; many physicians use the nurse as a means of arguing with other physicians. This places the nurse in an awkward, and often, as in this case, hostile position Physicians not only need to communicate in a professional manner with the nurses, they also need to communicate with each other and not use the nurse to pass messages to other physicians.

All licensed health care providers have had classes on theories of human behavior. Unfortunately, once they are out of school, they often forget what they have learned. The fact is that many educated people can act very uneducated when it comes to dealing with co-workers and other colleagues. The Theory of Mutual Respect and Collaboration is intended to remind those health care professionals how to conduct themselves on a professional level, and how to interact with others in an appropriate manner.

In most work places there are zero tolerance policies on aggression and intimidation. When a nurse or physician is rude and difficult to work with, this behavior disrupts the healing environment most health care facilities strive to create for patients. When this happens some facilities may take drastic action such as termination of employees who are difficult to work with or who are rude to others. Not only are hospitals and health care facilities transitioning to a more collaborative staff, the patients are demanding a peaceful environment in which to heal and recover as well. All it takes is a little effort on the part of the physician and nurse to make healthcare facilities places where the staff are respectful to each other and can collaborate with each other for the common good of the patient.

We have given some stories from the perspectives of patients and nurses; now we will give some stories from physician's perspectives. This is done to help readers gain insight into each view of a situation that could have had a different outcome had the Theory of Mutual Respect and Collaboration been utilized.

Nurse Know it All

"I had started working at five a.m. that morning, and I was very tired. I made rounds at multiple hospitals, and then went to my office to see patients in the clinic. I was on call that night as well and covering those same multiple hospitals. The beeper went off at two a.m. the next morning; I was asleep after such a long hectic day. The nurse who had paged me stated that the patient had

not produced any urine for the last 2-3 hours; he had only produced about 10-20cc for the last 24 hours. The nurse insisted that the patient needed diuretics; I did not want to give the patient diuretics because of his kidney function. The nurse kept persisting about the diuretics. I was half asleep and tired of arguing with her, so I agreed to give the order for the diuretics to help improve the patient's output. The next day the patient's kidney function was worse. The patient became dehydrated after the diuretics and ended up getting a fluid bolus. The lesson for me was to always investigate further, and not be badgered into giving an order just because a nurse thinks that it is the best course of action, and I don't want to argue anymore."
-Overworked and On Call Doctor

In this scenario the situation is turned and the nurse is the one who refuses to accept the input from the physician. Many nurses do have a high level of knowledge when it comes to patient care, but when a physician has just cause for ordering or not ordering some type of treatment, then the nurse should likewise be as respectful of the physician as he or she would want to be respected by the physician. The patient ultimately suffered because of the lack of respect the nurse had for the physician's expertise. Instead of arguing with the physician, the nurse would have benefitted from inquiring as to why the physician did not want to order the diuretics. Once the doors of communication and collaboration were opened, then the patient would not have had to suffer from dehydration induced because of a failure to collaborate on the nurse's part.

A Nurse's Judgment Call, You Be the Judge

"I was called by a nurse about a patient who had fallen. I instructed the nurse to get a CT scan of the head and an x-ray of the hip and back, then to call me with the results. When the nurse did call me, she told me the patient's condition had deteriorated. I went to see the patient and found her on a ventilator. I asked the nurse about the results of the head CT. She informed me that she did not get a CT of the head as was ordered, but just got an x-ray of the head because the CT was very expensive, and the patient had not hit her head anyway. The patient was very unstable at this time, so I said I wanted a CT of the head now. When the CT was done, it was discovered that the patient had a brain bleed. I was furious that a nurse took it upon herself to not do a test that I had specifically ordered. I did report her to administration, but I was exceptionally upset that this patient had a delay in treatment because of this nurse not doing what was ordered"   *-Anonymous Physician*

In this scenario the nurse was at fault for the delay in treatment because she did not follow the physician's instructions on patient care. In the Theory of Mutual Respect and Collaboration the nurse should have discussed the issue of the head CT with the physician at the time of the order. It is never a safe practice to dismiss a physician's order as unnecessary and to simply not carry them out. As a result of the nurse's failure to collaborate in the plan of care, the patient suffered harm.

Charged Up Nurse

"I was about to do surgery on a patient one day when a nurse caused the whole procedure to be stopped. The patient was on the operating room table for the procedure, scrubbed and with conscious sedation started. The nurse saw some EKG changes on the monitor and started shouting that the patient was having ventricular tachycardia and needed to be shocked. I looked at the patient who was still awake and talking and denying feeling anything different. The vital signs were stable, so I said, "It is okay." The nurse insisted we call a code and opened the code cart and was preparing to start shocking the patient. I stopped the procedure and said, "Get a cardiologist in here." A cardiologist, who was in house, came and reviewed the EKG strip that the nurse insisted was ventricular tachycardia and laughed and said it was just artifact. The patient had to be rescheduled for the procedure because we had wasted so much time on proving to the nurse that the patient was not coding, that our allotted time for the surgery was up, and we had to vacate the room for the next case." -*Anonymous Physician*

To call a code or not call a code; that was the question, but in this case was handled very poorly. In this scenario the nurse was not willing to communicate with the physician, even though the physician had a higher level of expertise. The physician did act appropriately by proving that the patient was not in a code situation. The nurse should have been willing to collaborate with the physician on whether the patient was truly in a lethal rhythm or not, but she was not. Her refusal to collaborate cost the staff and patient time and money. It is crucial for health care staff to be able to accept one another's contributions as valid. In this scenario the physician accepted the nurse's concerns about the EKG changes, but the nurse did not accept the physician's expertise in the care of the patient even though the physician gave valid reasons to proceed.

5. RESPECT

There are many definitions of respect; some consider it a courtesy toward others, while others show respect only to those whom they deem worthy of it. As healthcare professionals respect is something that needs to be shown to each other and to the patient. As professionals nurses and physicians need to show respect to each other especially in front of patients and visitors. Being respectful to other healthcare professionals can be difficult at times. When one healthcare professional is being disrespectful to another, the first thing the recipient wants to do is to retaliate and be disrespectful in return. This is another area where change in the healthcare profession needs to take place. Instead of reacting to someone's rude actions with more rudeness, professionals should maintain self-control and refrain from displaying the same ill mannerisms that were shown to them. If nurses and physicians can realize that their actions cause reactions from others and these reactions can be good or bad, then they may consider their actions more carefully before displaying them.

The way a message is conveyed can be perceived as disrespectful. Even if one person has caused another person to become upset, will it do any good to react with the same disrespect? It is much more professional use a calm tone in order to keep the situation from escalating. When tempers get out of control, this can escalate to a much harsher disagreement, so maintaining a calm tone, and showing a willingness to rectify the situation helps improve the chance of resolving the situation. It is human nature to become angry if we think we are being challenged or provoked. Instead of responding to rude actions by arguing back or being rude too, healthcare professionals should consider the end to this situation. They should ask themselves, "How will my reactions be interpreted, and how can this situation be resolved in a professional manner?" If these questions are considered prior to reacting to someone else's actions, then most likely the situation is already on the way to being resolved.

In the Theory of Mutual Respect and Collaboration this respect of others is a vital key to gaining respect in return. When others see healthcare professionals behaving with respect toward each other, they will want to show respect to others as well. Even when a person who has a lower level of education and/or intelligence is being disrespectful, it is important to always show that person respect; it does not help to insult that person's circumstance. Likewise if a person of higher education and socioeconomic status is rude and disrespectful, it does not improve the situation to also be rude.

When dealing with a rude person, it would be more dignified for the recipient of the rude behavior to maintain his or her composure and respond in a professional, calm manner. This reaction to the rude behavior will garner respect because the unprofessional behavior was met with professionalism. This book is not suggesting a person must accept rude behavior or be embarrassed or intimidated by others. On the contrary, it is the intent of this book to help individuals deal with unprofessional behavior in a professional manner. There are ways to voice your opinion, or disagreements with others without resorting to rude behavior.

Diva Doctor

"I remember one time I was working on a Sunday. One of the doctors had to come in and perform a procedure on a patient. He was not happy at all because he had to come in on the weekend, and he was very hateful. When he had finished, he told us to make sure his equipment was returned to his department. I was actually trying to be nice to him, so while he was documenting what he had done, I gathered his equipment and took it to him and said, "Here is your equipment; you can take it back with you, so it does not get lost." He became very red in the face and said, "Who do you think you are? I am not going to take this stuff myself." I said, "I'm sorry I thought you wanted to make sure it went back where it belongs." I really did not mean any disrespect to him at all. I don't know if he was just mad over having to come in on the weekend or something else, but he went from being offended to being enraged at me. He stood up and clinched his fist and told me I needed to know my role. Again, I apologized and said, "I will take care of the equipment." He started saying rude comments about how stupid nurses were and other things I can't remember. I do remember how embarrassed I was that he was acting this way in front of patients and visitors, but instead of blowing up at him, I walked away and took the equipment to the back of the unit. I came back up front and sat down on the other side of the unit. I was determined to not let this situation get out of control.

The doctor proceeded to come over to where I sat and started fussing again. I stood up and said, "I apologize again, and I will make sure your equipment is returned on Monday," and I walked away and headed to the bathroom where I knew he could not follow me. I stayed in there about fifteen minutes, and when I came out, he was gone. My co-worker was shocked at his behavior and also that I did not argue. I told him I was not going to act unprofessionally in front of patients. What I did do is a write him up for his disrespect toward me and his unprofessional behavior in front of patients. He never apologized to me, but he never talked to me that way again. Now whenever he passes me in the hall, he smiles and asks me how I am doing.

I did get ticked at him one day after that. I was sitting at the desk writing up another nurse (it was a have-to case); the report slips were on pink paper, so everyone knew when someone was writing someone up. He came in and saw the pink paper, and his eyes got big. I smiled and said, "Relax it is not you." He smiled, wiped his forehead, and laughed." -*Anonymous Nurse*

In this scenario even though the nurse may have wanted to retaliate against the physician's behavior, she remained calm and did not make the situation worse. She did make her feelings known to the physician in a professional manner that garnered respect instead of resentment. Too many times when a person is displaying disrespectful behavior toward someone, it is not meant to be a personal assault on that person; the person was the one at hand when the disruptive behavior erupted. If healthcare professionals can learn to not take rude behavior personally and instead look past it to find a professional solution to the problem, the outcome is better for everyone. It does not matter what provoked a person to be disrespectful; what matters is how the people around that person responds to it. The situation is almost similar to a heated political debate. The person who can stay calm and not give into the provocation of argument is usually the one who gains the most respect and gets the most votes. When respect is shown to others, it will certainly be returned, maybe not immediately but eventually.

There are many reasons why someone may exhibit rude or disrespectful behavior. He or she could be having any number of problems associated with everyday life. When a person cannot separate personal life from the professional one, emotions can lead to irrational behaviors. This is not to say this behavior is acceptable, but if we can understand why someone is behaving in an unprofessional way, then we will not be as quick to act the same way.

Respect is something that everyone needs. According to Abraham Maslow, esteem has two essential components. One is the respect of others and the other is self-respect. When people have self-respect and the respect of others, they are more effective in their lives and jobs. If a person is treated disrespectfully, this decreases self-respect and confidence. An employee who feels intimidated or threatened may perform poorly. Working under intimidating or hostile conditions is not conducive to optimal performance. This creates a decrease in employee satisfaction, and this dis-satisfaction can spill over to feelings of low self- esteem.

When disrespect is shown to someone it creates a block to effective communication. This does not promote progress toward a common goal of effective patient care and outcomes. Consideration should be made as to why disrespectful actions occur. Does it make the perpetrator feel more empowered to treat others rudely or unprofessionally? If so, then there may be underlying causes to this person's disruptive behavior, and it may not have anything to do with the recipient of the behavior at all. In this case a rude, disrespectful person may want to consider his or her own faults before pointing out everyone else's.

Healthcare providers who are intimidated by others are more likely to make mistakes. According to a report from the National Academies, medical errors affect 1.5 million people and cost around 3.5 billion extra dollars annually. (Bootman, 2006) When a healthcare provider exhibits disrespectful behavior to others, it affects more than just that person's emotions. The end result of intimidation can be an expensive one. Because of the spiraling effects, rude and disrespectful behavior between healthcare providers can have astronomical physical and monetary consequences. This makes changing the relationship between the physician and nurse crucial. This behavior is not going to be tolerated by healthcare facilities, whether it is nurses who disrespect each other, or physicians who disrespect others, employers will make the necessary changes to encourage respect and professionalism in the workplace. With today's healthcare reform, healthcare organizations will get paid for performance. If that performance is impeded because nurses or physicians do not maintain professional behavior, then the organization may be forced to release the disruptive party from employment. There have been stories that have circulated about nurses being afraid to ask or tell a physician anything because that particular physician was considered mean or cruel. Likewise some nurses have built a reputation of being argumentative and unapproachable. These types of employees will become unemployed as well if they do not change or modify their behavior in the workplace; healthcare organizations cannot afford to keep employees such as these.

Respect for other cultures is also a requirement in the healthcare field. The world is becoming smaller as people are interacting more globally than they did in the past. Healthcare providers have to be aware of other cultures and be able to show respect for other's beliefs. This is not to say a person has to disregard his or her own beliefs, but it is possible to work with other cultures in a professional manner while maintaining one's own beliefs. Healthcare has become so multicultural that it is impossible not to work at some point with someone who has a different cultural background than yours. This should be viewed as an opportunity, not an obstacle to collaboration. Too many times nurses and physicians get so stuck in their own ways of doing things that it is almost as if they are going around with blinders on. Because diversity is constantly increasing in the healthcare field, communication and collaboration among nurses and physicians becomes increasingly important.

6. COLLABORATION

Traditionally collaboration between physicians and nurses consisted of the physician giving orders which the nurses followed. This practice is still widely followed today; the difference is that patients and nurses have access to more information than ever before, and with this increased level of knowledge and education patients and nurses are taking a more active role in the plan of care. Also nurses are required to maintain a higher level of training in their area of expertise. There are different areas of practice such as cardiology, obstetrics, orthopedics, and neurology. Nurses working in these areas are required to maintain higher credentialing to keep their jobs. Since nurses are required to maintain a certain level of expertise in their field of practice, they are held more accountable for their actions or inactions regarding patient care. There are lawsuits in the court system these days that argue that nurses are just as responsible in medical malpractice suits as the physicians, when they see a physician doing something wrong. The suits contend that the nurses had a high level of education and expertise in that area and should be held as accountable as the physicians because they did not intervene on the patient's behalf. The change in legal perceptions of the roles and accompanying accountability is another reason attitudes need to change. Since the nurse is being considered an expert by the court systems, the physician also must place value on the nurse's contribution of information as well.

The traditional roles of physician and nurses are no longer an acceptable practice in modern medicine. This is where the Theory of Mutual Respect and Collaboration can help physicians and nurses as they transition into a new more collaborative relationship in which both contribute information that is accepted by the other. For this reason it is imperative for physicians and nurses to show respect and professional courtesy toward each other; then effective collaboration can take place. The common goal is to improve patient outcomes, so it is not a question of if this new role transition takes place; it is a question of when it will take place. Healthcare has always been a changing field, and the relationship between the physicians and nurses, as well as the patient, is changing too. Healthcare practitioners from all areas have to work together; the trends in healthcare today demand collaboration between the patient, nurse, and physician. This is not about dissolving the traditional hierarchy, but closing the gaps in communication.

Collaboration Saved Christmas

"I remember taking care of a little elderly lady two days before Christmas. She was supposed to be discharged that day. The cardiology group had signed off on her, but her heart rate would drop down into the forties. Although she was not symptomatic, I was still concerned about her going home with her heart rate dropping like that. The cardiology group said it was fine because she was not showing any symptoms associated with bradycardia. I called her primary doctor to let him know that cardiology said she could go home. I also discussed with him how the patient's heart rate had dropped. I suggested to him that we keep her one more day. He agreed with me and thanked me for my input. About three hours later the patient's heart actually stopped, and we had to perform CPR on her. She ended up with a temporary pacemaker and had a permanent one put in the next day. I am glad the primary doctor worked with me on this patient since otherwise she may have died at home that day. "

-Anonymous Nurse

In this scenario, the physician collaborated with the nurse for the good of the patient. There was mutual respect shown for each provider's information, and the patient's outcome was improved through collaboration between the physician and the nurse.

Getting To the Heart of the Matter

"I was recently taking care of a patient complaining of chest pain who had been transferred to our facility from a small outlying hospital because we had a cardiac program. The patient arrived, and we did a series of tests to rule out myocardial infarction. We did lab work and EKGs on the patient to compare to tests from the other hospital. The patient did not complain of chest pain upon arriving at our hospital, nor were there any EKG changes noted, and the cardiac enzymes were within normal limits. The cardiologist who was consulted came in to evaluate the patient who had elevated enzymes and was having chest pain and the accompanying report given to him by the transferring physician. The cardiologist was in the process of preparing to take the patient to the catheter lab because he thought the patient might be having a heart attack. I asked the physician to take a look at the patient's EKGs and labs. He did and also noted that there had been no changes, and the labs were within normal limits. The physician told me he was given the understanding the patient could be infarcting, and thanked me for calling his attention to this. He told me I saved the patient from having an unnecessary procedure. " -*Critical Care Nurse.*

In this scenario the physician was willing to accept the information contributed by the nurse. Even though he had received a report from the transferring physician, he listened to the information the nurse had to offer, and this contributed to the effective collaboration of caring for the patient. Likewise the collaboration between the physician and the nurse prevented the patient from undergoing unnecessary treatment. This saved the patient time and money from a prolonged hospital stay.

GI Bleeding Blues

"I was working in the cardiac unit, and I assumed care of a patient who had been admitted the night before. The night shift nurse had given me the report, and the plan was to do a cardiac work up because the patient had been discharged just three days prior to this recent admission. The patient had just had stents placed, so naturally the idea was that the patient was having cardiac problems. When I assessed the patient, he told me did not have any chest pain at all, just stomach pain. I reviewed the patient's lab work, and it revealed a low blood count. The blood count was not critically low, but I reviewed the labs from the prior admission to compare the two. There had been a significant drop. When the cardiologist arrived, I gave this information to him. We sent stools for occult blood and discovered the patient had a GI bleed, so instead of getting a cardiac work up that he did not need, a gastroenterologist was consulted and that doctor managed the GI bleed. The cardiologist was thankful and so was the patient that we did not waste time on a cardiology work up, and possibly put the patient at risk for a worsening bleed from the blood thinners that accompany a cardiac workup." -*Anonymous Nurse*

In this scenario the nurse had a knowledge base that guided her to check for other possible causes of the illness. When a nurse presents information to a physician, that physician has the choice to listen to it or dismiss it. In this case if the physician had dismissed the information and proceeded with the cardiac work up, the patient could have endured serious consequences from the blood thinners used in the cardiac work up. The collaboration between the physician and the nurse prevented a serious health complication for the patient. Also, had the nurse not offered this information and the physician proceeded with the cardiac work up, and the patient had developed serious complications or death as a result, it would have been very difficult to figure out what had happened. A small amount of collaboration can go a long way in ensuring the safety of a patient, and it is definitely worth the effort of both nurses and physicians to share information with each other.

7. RESOLUTION

There are scenarios when immediate resolution cannot be found. When this occurs, there are usually facility policies to handle disagreements, such as a chain of command. This usually involves a hierarchy of employee, immediate supervisor, director, human resource director, CEO, and/or a grievance committee. These steps are in place to help employees have a way to handle their differences in a professional manner. The problem is that many people do not want to take a disagreement to this level for fear of repercussions. This is when some people try to handle things on their own, and the situation can worsen dramatically for the person. If there is someone who displays rude behavior and refuses to try to modify his or her behavior to be more professional, then following the chain of command is the best practice to help educate that person regarding how to be professional. Remember, maintaining a respectful, professional behavior does not mean letting others treat you rudely; quite the opposite. The Theory of Mutual Respect and Collaboration is meant to help individuals learn how to conduct themselves as professionals and teach others to do the same. Most organizations have policies regarding expected behavior from employees. This is not to say disagreements will not arise in the work place because they will. The Theory of Mutual Respect and Collaboration is a tool to help resolve the issue in a more professional manner.

Dr. My Way or the Highway

"I had been working in a hospital for many years as a physician. The doctors and nurses had always had very congenial relationships. Then the hospital hired a physician who wanted to prove that nobody else knew as much as he did. Many of the nurses were told by him to not be around him when he was seeing his patients. He told the nursing staff they were stupid and did not know how to take care of patients. One day this doctor called me and told me not to write orders on patients he was following. I explained to him that I was also following some of the same patients as a consult. He stated he did not agree with my orders; I informed him that I was using evidence based practice. He said he did not care about evidence based practice; I was not to write orders. I could not reason with him because he refused to listen to reason. I went to the Medical Director about the situation. The doctor was so unreasonable that he was fired and his contract was terminated." *-Anonymous Doctor*

These Boots Are Made For Walking

"I used to have a supervisor who for some reason did not care for me at all and made no effort to hide the fact. After many confrontations and frequent rude interactions, I asked that person why I was being treated that way. The reply was that we had strong personalities that clashed. I admit that I have a strong personality; if someone accuses me of something I did not do, I will vehemently defend myself. When I could not get anything resolved with that manager, I went up the chain of command. This did not resolve the problem either. Eventually I decided the best thing to do was to switch departments. At first I felt as if I were being forced out of a position that I loved, then I soon came to realize that from the constant arguing with that manager I had been under a lot of stress. I did not realize how much stress I was under until I left. Now that I am away from all the chaos, I do not feel that I lost the battle; I feel I won the war."

-Disgruntled Employee

In these scenarios, although resolution could not be gained through the chain of command, there was a way to get past it. Sometimes people fail to try to get resolution because they think it makes them appear weak, when, on the contrary, it is better to walk away from a situation that cannot be resolved in a professional manner. The key point is to remain professional even when others are not.

Often resolution cannot be achieved because one person is not willing to compromise for fear of seeming like a push over or a weak person. If all parties involved looked at the problem from an objective point of view, they might be able to see the opposing side. It is easier to resolve conflicts if the other side of the problem is understood, but too often people will not even attempt to see the problem from another's point of view. This is one of the reasons it is sometimes impossible to resolve workplace disagreements.

Many situations can be resolved long before they ever become a problem. This can be done by simply asking ourselves before we speak, "Is what I am about to say going to help or hurt the situation?" The age old advice of "Think before you speak" is still very applicable today. We may also ask ourselves, "How can I say what I want to say without being derogatory to the other person?" It is possible to make your point and say what you want to say, and still remain professional. When a person makes a statement or displays an action that causes another to be angry or upset, instead of letting human nature get the upper hand and retaliating, it is far more beneficial for both parties to refrain from lashing out. Resolution can be found if each person keeps an open mind and respectful attitude. This may be hard to do, especially when someone has a short temper to begin with. It takes time to master self-control in these situations. The main thing to remember is that in the health care profession, maintaining professionalism in any situation is not only beneficial to the employees, but also to the patients.

Nurse Pushy Pants

"When I had just begun my nursing career, there was an older nurse who had a reputation for being mean to new nurses; she was very pushy and bossy. Back then we had to count the medication carts; there were only four carts and five nurses. This meant that two of the nurses had to share a cart. It was kind of a silent rule that whoever counted the cart was the one who got to use it. I finished up reports, and the night shift nurse wanted to know who was going to count the cart with her. I looked at the older nurse who kept looking down at her report sheets and did not respond, so I told the night shift nurse that I would count with her. I finished counting and was getting my report sheets and medication lists in order when the older nurse came up to me and said, "Give me the keys to my cart." I replied, "I counted it, so I am using it." She retorted, "That is my cart and I don't care if you did count it. Give me the keys." Since she was used to bullying the other nurses and getting her way, she thought she could do that with me. I told her "No" and that she would have to share a cart with someone else. She became very angry and said, "I am going to get the charge nurse, and then you will have to give me the keys". She did get the charge nurse and returned. She told the charge nurse that I had the keys to her cart and would not give them to her. She also said, "She is new around here, (referring to me) and you need to straighten her out on how things work." The charge nurse looked at me, and before she could say anything, I said, "From what I understand whoever counts the cart gets to use it. I gave her time to get up and count the cart, but she didn't. I counted the cart and now she wants to take it away from me." The charge nurse asked the older nurse, "Did she count the cart?" The older nurse answered, "Yes, but it doesn't matter." The charge nurse said, "Oh yes, it does." I got to keep the cart that day. The older nurse was mad the rest of the day, and for the rest of the time I worked there she did not speak to me or try to bully me for that matter. I did not act unprofessionally toward her, but I did stand my ground with her and this brought resolution to my situation."   -*Anonymous Nurse*

In this scenario an older, more experienced nurse used intimidation of new nurses to show her authority. The difference was this particular new nurse was not intimidated and used the silent rule to her advantage, while remaining professional. When another staff member tries to use bullying or intimidation as a means to get what he or she wants, there are ways to resolve the issue without resorting to the same tactics. In this case the charge nurse played a key role in doing the right thing, by allowing the new nurse to keep the cart for the day. If employees are trying to do the right thing and another staff member tries to misuse his or her seniority or position to take advantage of someone else, there are rules in place in most facilities to avoid or resolve these situations. (Bootman, 2006)

In the Theory of Mutual respect and Collaboration resolutions to problems do not just pertain to the health care field. This theory can be used in many different areas of life.

Mr. Mizer

"I was in the grocery store line, and an elderly gentleman was in front of me. The cashier totaled up his items and told him how much it was. He asked her how much he had been charged for a package of meat, and she told him. He told her that was too much; he said there was a sign that listed it as $2.59 a pound, but the computer was charging more for it. The cashier was polite, and the gentleman was frank but not rude. She went to find out the correct price. She did not find out the correct price, so she just gave the man the discounted price, and he left without even saying thank you. As soon as he was out the door, another employee came to the register with the right price; it was more than the $2.59; it was $3.99. The sign was between two different packages of meat. The cashier said I wished I had known that because I would not have given him the sale price because he was not nice at all. I looked at her and said, "Honey just consider the source. He is an old man on a fixed income and every penny counts." She smiled and replied, "You're right."

-Anonymous Shopper

Resolution

In this scenario the Theory of Mutual Respect worked because in the end the cashier did consider the life and situation of the customer. When people encounter situations where there could be disagreements or arguments, they need to consider the other person's circumstances. This can help resolve the situation by providing a rationale for the other person's behavior. If one person disregards the circumstances of another, often a resolution cannot be achieved because there will be no insight as to why that person is behaving the way he or she is. This theory can be used by anyone in any situation to help bring resolution to sometimes difficult situations.

Patients, physicians, and nurses all have an increased level of knowledge now. They all should understand that with this increase in knowledge comes greater responsibility. This new knowledge must be used responsibly. As health care providers try to formulate a holistic plan of care for the patient, they must each take an active role while being respectful of others' contributions. There often are multiple ways of achieving a goal or performing a job. If a physician or nurse thinks that something is not being done correctly, both have a responsibility to collaborate with the other to achieve the best possible outcome for the patient. As can be seen in the scenarios we have provided, when any member of the health care team, including the patient, refuses to collaborate, the patient usually suffers, but the medical organization and all of its employees may suffer also.

The stories we have shared in this book have illustrated various degrees of collaboration failure and success. As with any problem there are solutions, so next we will present ways to help resolve collaboration issues in the health care field.

If a patient does not agree with the physician's treatment plan, he or she has a right to get a second opinion. The physician or nurse should not take offense to this, but instead should offer to help the patient gain as much knowledge and information about the disease process as possible. If this means referring the patient to another physician, then that is what needs to be done. Likewise if physicians and nurses have disagreements about what needs to be done in a plan of care, instead of behaving in an unprofessional manner toward each other, each should support his or her decisions with valid research and a great deal of experience. This will open the lines of communication and improve collaboration, further strengthening all of the healthcare team dynamics.

8. FUTURE OF HEALTH CARE

As was shown earlier, the roles of the patient, nurse, and physician have changed over the years. The current and future technology will enhance the expertise of the patient, nurse, and physician. All three will have access to peer-reviewed reports and articles on any given health care disease or illness. Many patients and nurses will educate themselves on particular diseases, treatments, and medications in order to manage the problem more effectively. When caring for a patient that has a disease or illness with which the nurse is not familiar, that nurse can gain knowledge by using many different web sites that have detailed information about caring for a patient with that particular problem. Patients can also become very knowledgeable about their own diseases by researching databases on the internet that have information specifically for them, so it is easier to understand. Health Care Reform is also a major influence that will be changing the health care field. In the push for universal healthcare, there is also a push for health care organizations to update their software systems; with this advancement in networking, the access to health information will be even more readily available to patients, nurses, and physicians.

The role of nurses is still changing and evolving. Many nurses now have also obtained business degrees and are serving on hospital boards, as CEOs of organizations, and on national-level policy boards. With these new roles in healthcare, many nurses and physicians have developed much closer working relationships. Although the roles of the nurse and physician are different, they are of equal importance in the provision of healthcare. In the healthcare reform overhaul, there is a collaborative effort between policy makers, healthcare leaders, and health care providers to decrease the unnecessary waste in providing healthcare. For this reason nurses and physicians alike are being asked to contribute new ideas regarding how to reduce spending. The focus is on reducing waste while maintaining quality health care. Input from all areas of healthcare is readily accepted as health care leaders and politicians strive to develop new policies and create a more cost effective, patient centered, and high quality system.

It is the intention of this book to make physicians and nurses realize they have to work together in order to prevent chaos. The goal is not to cause the physician to relinquish authority regarding patient care to nurses, but quite the contrary. Physicians must realize that nurses, as well as patients, have a knowledge base of their own and can contribute valuable information to the plan of care. Likewise nurses need to realize that although physicians do have a higher level of education than they do, the contribution of information made by nurses is equally important in developing a plan of care for the patient and working toward the common goal of getting the patient back to an optimal state of health. The Theory of Mutual Respect and Collaboration is a tool to help individuals work more effectively with each other. This theory is not limited to the health care field. People from any line of work can apply this theory to their everyday lives in order to interact with others in a positive way.

9. THEORY OF MUTUAL RESPECT AND COLLABORATION

In the age of modern technology and health care reform, consumers are demanding to be part of the decision making process as well as expecting collaboration between those who provide health care services to them. It is imperative that health care providers work together for the common good of the patient. One way to do this is for nurses and physicians to understand each other in a more holistic way, so they can work more effectively together. The Theory of Mutual Respect and Collaboration is intended to help the key people that create the fundamental dynamics involved in providing health care to understand that each individual does have something unique to offer. All people are individuals with a certain knowledge base and valuable abilities. All must show a certain amount of acceptance and compassion toward others and be able to respect others and themselves. In the theory, if each person explores the areas of uniqueness while recognizing the areas of common interest, they will be able to work together effectively. The theory was developed in the hope that health care providers would start working together in a more collaborative way and improve the way health care is delivered. When everyone works together the result will be improved outcomes for patients and more efficient and effective relationships among health care system.

REFERENCES

(1) Furberg, C.D., A. A. Levin, P.A. Gross, R. S. Shapiro, and B.L.Strom. 2006 The FDA and Drug Safety: A Proposal for Sweeping Changes. ARCH Intern Med 166(18):1938-42

(2) Gordon S. Antibiotics Still Prescribed To Often, includes interview with expert Dr. Philip Tierno, originally published by Health Day News, November 8, 2005, reprinted by PharmDaily.Com.http://www.pharndaily.com/Article/1722/Antibiotics_Still_Prescribed_Too_Oftenhtml?CategoryID=29

(3) Gurwitz, J. H., T. S. Field, J. Avorn, D. McCormick, S. Jain, M. Eckler, M. Benser, A. C. Edmondson, and D. W. Bates. 2000. Incidence and preventability of adverse drug events in nursing homes. Am J Med 109(2):87-94

(4) Centers for Disease Control and Prevention. Estimates of Healthcare-Associated Infections, last modified May 30, 2007. http://www.cdc.gov/ncidod/dhqp/html

(5) US National Center for Health Statistics. Deaths: Final Data for 2005. National Vital Statistics Report, vol. 10, April 24, 2008.
http://www.cdc.gov/nchs/data/nvsr.nvsr56/nvsr5610.pdf

(6)Hospitals May Be Hazardous To Your Health. (2013, February 2).

(7) National Coalition of Health Care. Economic Cost Fact Sheets: The Impact of Rising Health Care Costs of the Economy, NCHC, 2009.
http://www.nchc.org/facts/economic.shtml

(8) Wyden, Ron Senator, The Healthy Americans Act.

"$2.2trillion currently spent of health care in America today."
http://wyden,senate.gov/issues/Legislation/Healthy_American _Act.cfm

(9) National Coalition on HealthCare. Health Insurance Costs: Facts on the Cost of Health Insurance and Health Care, NCHC, 2009. http://www.nchc.org/facts/cost.shtml

(10) National Coalition on HealthCare. "Did You Know?" section of home page of NCHC, 2009
http://www.nchc.org/

(11) Sexton at al: Error, Stress, and Teamwork in Medicine and Aviation: Cross sectional surveys Sexton at al: BMJ V.320(7237);March 18,2000

ABOUT THE AUTHORS

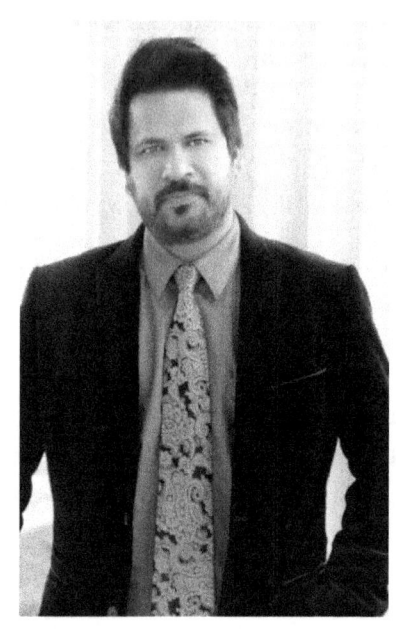

Kamran Hasni, M.D., graduated from Dow Medical College in Karachi, Pakistan and completed his residency in internal medicine at Drexel University in Philadelphia, where he also completed his Fellowship in Nephrology. Dr. Hasni is board certified in Internal Medicine and Nephrology, and has practiced medicine in different settings from big city hospitals to rural health facilities. Dr. Hasni has published numerous abstracts and papers. He has also published the first DVD on Interventional Nephrology Real time curriculum. As community based Associate Professor of Medicine at the University of Kentucky, College of Medicine, and an Adjunct faculty at Lincoln Memorial University, Dr. Hasni has extensive experience teaching medical students and nurses. Dr. Hasni was awarded the Compassionate Physician Award and On Time Doctor Award in 2009 and the Patient's Choice Award in 2008, 2009 and 2013.

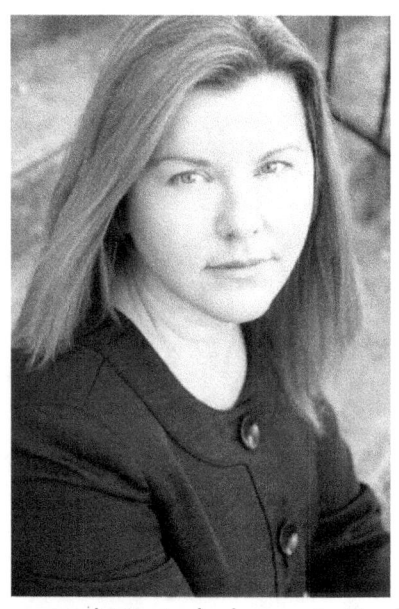

Mary Perkins R.N., M.S.N., M.H.A., completed her Associate Degree in Nursing at Lincoln Memorial University. After working in the field of nursing for 10 years as a staff nurse and preceptor to nursing students, she went on to obtain a BSN from the University of Phoenix. She has just completed a MSN and a second Master's degree in Health Care Administration. She plans to pursue a career in administration as well as teaching, while working toward her Doctorate in Nursing Practice. In her work as a patient care advocate, Mrs. Perkins has been awarded recognition as "Ambassador of Caring" for the hospital where she worked in 2005.

www.ingramcontent.com/pod-product-compliance
Lightning Source LLC
Chambersburg PA
CBHW051728170526
45167CB00002B/850